What you really need to know about

IRRITABLE BOWEL SYNDROME

Dr. Robert Buckman
with Nigel Howard

Introduced by John Cleese

LEBHAR-FRIEDMAN BOOKS

New York • Chicago • Los Angeles • London • Paris • Tokyo

Lebhar-Friedman Books
425 Park Avenue
New York, NY 10022

A Marshall Edition
Conceived by Marshall Editions
The Orangery
161 New Bond Street
London W1Y 9PA

First U.S. edition published 2000 by Lebhar-Friedman Books.

First published in the UK in 2000 by Marshall Publishing Ltd.
Copyright © 2000 Marshall Editions Developments Ltd.

Library of Congress Cataloging-in-Publication Data
on file at the Library of Congress

ISBN 0-86730-827-3

Originated in Italy by Articolor
Printed in and bound in Italy by Milanostampa

Managing Editor Theresa Reynolds
Art Editor Siân Keogh
U.S. Editor Maggi McCormick
Indexer Susan Bosanko
Illustrator Martin Laurie
Photographer Martin Norris
Series Managing Editor Anne Yelland
Managing Art Editor Helen Spencer
Editorial Director Ellen Dupont
Art Director Dave Goodman
D.T.P Editor Lesley Gilbert
Editorial Coordinator Ros Highstead
Production Nikki Ingram, Anna Pauletti

Cover photography: front Superstock; back Dick Luria/ Telegraph Colour Library

The consultant for this book was Shari Leipzig, M.D., who is an obstetrician and gynecologist in general practice in
New York City. She is also a clinical instructor of obstetrics and gynecology at Mt. Sinai School of Medicine.

Note: The words "he" and "she," used in alternate articles, are equally applicable to men and women.

Contents

Foreword

Most of you know me best as someone who makes people laugh.

But for 30 years I have also been involved with communicating information. And one particular area in which communication often breaks down is the doctor/patient relationship. We have all come across doctors who fail to communicate clearly, using complex medical terms when a simple explanation would do, and dismiss us with a "come back in a month if you still don't feel well." Fortunately, I met Dr. Robert Buckman.

Rob is one of North America's leading experts on cancer, but far more importantly he is a doctor who believes that hiding behind medical jargon is unhelpful and unprofessional. He wants his patients to understand what is wrong with them, and spends many hours with them—and their families and close friends—making sure they understand everything. Together we created a series of videos, with the jargon-free title *Videos for Patients*. Their success has prompted us to write books that explore medical conditions in the same clear, simple terms.

This book is one of a series that will tell you all you need to know about your condition. It assumes nothing. If you have a helpful, honest, communicative doctor, you will find here the extra information that he or she simply may not have time to tell you. If you are less fortunate, this book will help to give you a much clearer picture of your situation.

More importantly—and this was a major factor in the success of the videos—you can access the information here again and again. Turn back, read over, until you really know what your doctor's diagnosis means.

In addition, because in the middle of a consultation, you may not think of everything you would like to ask your doctor, you can also use the book to help you formulate the questions you would like to discuss with him or her.

John Cleese

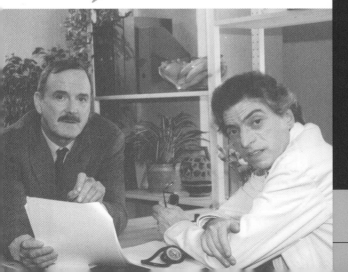

Introduction

DID YOU KNOW?

IBS affects people of all ages; symptoms usually appear between the ages of 20 and 45.

The exact cause of irritable bowel syndrome is still unknown.

As the title says, this book aims to tell you what you really need to know about an extremely common health problem, irritable bowel syndrome or IBS for short. It does not attempt to cram every last theory, piece of research, or diet fad between its covers. Instead, it cuts through the mass of confusing information that surrounds IBS to give you the basic facts about this distressing and often misunderstood condition.

How the book works

The book describes the symptoms of IBS, outlines what little is known about its causes, and explains how your doctor will go about making a diagnosis. It then goes on to show how, once you have been diagnosed as having IBS, you can take action to overcome the problem by making changes in your lifestyle.

Taking action

A few people with IBS are able to identify a particular trigger for their symptoms, such as a food to which they are sensitive, and avoid it. However, for most sufferers from IBS life is not that simple because the cause of their symptoms cannot be determined.

If you belong to this majority, don't despair. It may take longer, but as this book shows, there are still plenty of approaches that can help you reduce your symptoms in the long term, though you may not be able to eliminate them altogether.

If your symptoms are particularly troublesome, medical treatment from your doctor, explained in Chapter Two, will help, albeit as a short-term measure. Once your symptoms have been eased you can start looking for a way to reduce their frequency and severity.

Coping with the condition

Irritable bowel syndrome is what is known as a paroxysmal condition, which is a medical way of saying that it comes and goes, with the symptoms entirely absent at some times, then becoming very severe. The symptoms and severity of IBS vary considerably from person to person, but for most individuals the condition follows a pattern of rumbling along, causing the occasional problem, then flaring up for a while before subsiding again.

Obviously, the ideal solution is to find out what is triggering your symptoms. Some of the approaches explained in Chapter Three can help you do this. You can take steps to prevent your symptoms from flaring up again. Chapter Four looks at basic diet and lifestyle changes that can help you achieve this.

INTESTINAL DISEASE FOUNDATION

Founded in 1986, The Intestinal Disease Foundation seeks to help people improve their quality of life and better manage the everyday symptoms of chronic intestinal illnesses including irritable bowel syndrome. The organization conducts educational programs, organizes support groups, offers a telephone support network, and can make physician and dietician referrals.

Their quarterly newsletter *Intestinal Fortitude* contains articles by physicians, psychologists, pharmacists, dietitians, and other health-care professionals, and is free to members, of which there are currently 1,200. You can find contact details on page 78.

Chapter

1

SYMPTOMS &
CAUSES

What is IBS?

IBS affects about 20% of the adult population of the U.S.

Although IBS can be distressing, it is not a life-threatening disease.

Irritable bowel syndrome, or IBS for short, is an extremely common digestive disorder. Its symptoms can include abdominal pain, bloating, constipation, and diarrhea. The symptoms can be mild, or they can be serious enough to interfere with everyday life.

How serious is IBS?

IBS may be uncomfortable and unpleasant, but it is not life-threatening. However, it does share some symptoms with other, more serious disorders of the bowel such as ulcerative colitis (inflammation and ulceration of the large intestine) or Crohn's disease (inflammation of the lower part of the small intestine). It is therefore important to have your condition diagnosed by a doctor to exclude the possibility that you have one of these conditions.

How common is IBS?

If you have IBS, you are not alone. In the developed countries of the world between 10 and 22 percent of the population have symptoms of IBS at some time or another, and one in 10 people are affected seriously enough to seek medical help. Irritable bowel syndrome is the most common reason for people to see a gastroenterologist (a doctor who specializes in problems of the stomach and intestines), but less than 50% of people with IBS seek medical help.

Who suffers from IBS?

IBS affects people of all ages; symptoms usually first appear between the ages of 15 and 40. Twice as many women as men are affected, and women are also more likely to consult their doctor about symptoms. (This is not universal; in India, more men than women are affected.)

SOME COMMON MISCONCEPTIONS

MYTH	REALITY
"IBS IS HEREDITARY."	Other members of the family may have similar symptoms, but you do not have an increased risk of suffering from IBS just because your parents did.
"YOU CAN CATCH IBS FROM A BACTERIA OR VIRUS."	It is not caused by an infection from a bacteria or virus, although it can sometimes be triggered by a bout of "Montezuma's revenge" or gastroenteritis.
"ONCE YOU GET IBS, YOUR CONDITION WILL DETERIORATE OVER TIME."	IBS is not a progressive disorder; in other words, it does not get worse as time goes by. Instead, it is there, grumbling away in the background, occasionally flaring up and then subsiding.
"IBS IS NOT A REAL ILLNESS—IT'S ALL IN THE MIND."	Like many health problems, IBS can be made worse by stress and anxiety, but its symptoms result from a physical disorder.

YOU REALLY NEED TO KNOW

◆ IBS is a common digestive disorder affecting mainly young and middle-aged adults, though it can occur at any age.

◆ Symptoms may be mild, and not all sufferers seek a doctor's help.

◆ IBS is not life-threatening, infectious, progressive, or all in the mind.

What is IBS?

Symptoms of IBS

✓ Many people suffer some of the symptoms of IBS from time to time, but don't have the syndrome.

✗ IBS sufferers experience symptoms over a long period of time—occasional bouts of constipation, diarrhea, or abdominal pain don't amount to IBS.

Irritable bowel syndrome is not a disease in the true sense of the word. It is a condition or disorder. "Syndrome" is the medical term for a group of symptoms that often occur together and are associated with a single disorder.

The symptoms of IBS vary between individuals and from time to time. Some people experience an occasional abdominal pain and need to rush to the bathroom first thing in the morning to empty their bowels, while others suffer the full range of symptoms. All those with IBS will experience some or all of the symptoms discussed here.

Abdominal pain or discomfort

This can be experienced either as a continuous dull ache or in the form of cramps, both of which come and go in waves. Pain and discomfort can occur anywhere in the

WHAT DOES IT MEAN?

CONSTIPATION

Constipation is usually defined as having a bowel movement less than three times a week or straining to pass stools (feces) or a sense of incomplete emptying.

DIARRHEA

Diarrhea is defined as a loose consistency of stool with more than three bowel movements daily lasting longer than two weeks.

SYNDROME

A collection of symptoms that often occur together and are associated with a single disorder.

abdominal area, although it tends to be worse low down on the left-hand side. The pain generally comes on after eating and is worse during bouts of constipation. It is frequently relieved by opening the bowels or by passing gas.

Bloating

IBS sufferers often experience feelings of abdominal bloating, so that clothes feel tight and uncomfortable. The bloating sensation may be accompanied by rumbling noises and flatulence (gas). It is often triggered by eating and may get worse over the course of a day.

Constipation and diarrhea

Of the two, constipation is more common in IBS sufferers, though sometimes constipation and diarrhea alternate in the same individual. These symptoms are often accompanied by pain. In some people diarrhea comes on after a meal or when they wake up in the morning, and the need to empty the bowels may be so urgent that they cannot reach the toilet in time.

Other changes in the stools

Stools can become small, hard, and pelletlike, and can be covered in mucus—the mucous glands in the bowel walls become overstimulated by prolonged contact with slow-moving stools. It is not uncommon just to pass mucus.

A feeling of incomplete emptying

After going to the toilet, sufferers from IBS may still feel they need to empty their bowels. This can lead to ineffective straining to pass further stools and may trigger a sharp, cramping pain deep in the rectum (back passage).

YOU REALLY NEED TO KNOW

◆ IBS is not a disease, it is a condition or disorder.

◆ Symptoms vary from person to person and from time to time.

◆ Sufferers from IBS may experience only some of the symptoms mentioned.

Symptoms of IBS

Related problems

Sometimes IBS symptoms can lead to further problems. Constantly straining to pass stools because of constipation, for example, can lead to hemorrhoids (piles). IBS sufferers often experience other disorders which, although not directly caused by their bowel problems, are thought to be related to the syndrome.

Anal fissure

Very large, hard stools can tear the anal canal lining as they pass through, especially if they are passed quickly. There is usually some pain as the stool is passed, a little

HEMORRHOIDS (PILES)

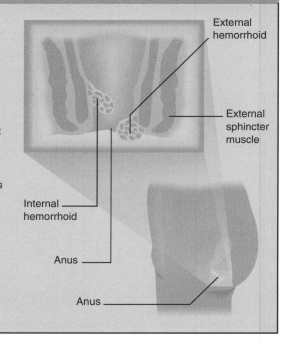

Straining to pass stools due to constipation may damage the veins in and around the anus; the valves give way, and the veins become dilated (this is exactly what happens with varicose veins in the legs). A soft lump forms that may feel uncomfortable, though rarely painful. Hemorrhoids, or piles, may develop inside the anus or on its outer edge. They may be damaged and bleed when stools pass over them. If the blood trapped in an external pile clots, the pile may become extremely painful. A doctor can anesthetize the area and remove the clot.

External hemorrhoid

External sphincter muscle

Internal hemorrhoid

Anus

Anus

bleeding, and more pain on passing stools subsequently. The pain can make the sufferer delay passing stools, which makes constipation worse.

The tear may heal of its own accord within a few days; if not, a doctor can prescribe a local anesthetic cream to numb the area until it does. A chronic fissure may require treatment under general anesthesia.

Other symptoms

IBS sufferers commonly experience non-intestinal symptoms. The range is wide: fatigue and lethargy, urinary frequency and urgency, recurrent back and loin pain, painful sexual intercourse, chest pain and palpitations, shortness of breath, wheezing, and hyperventilation have all been reported. This has led sufferers in the past to be dismissed as hypochondriacs, or to be misdiagnosed.

Research has confirmed, however, that IBS sufferers are more likely to develop some of these symptoms throughout their life. They are also more likely to develop asthma. One study found that 22.4 percent of IBS sufferers had over-sensitive lung airways, compared with only 12.2 percent in nonsufferers.

Anxiety and depression

IBS may be accompanied by anxiety and depression in some sufferers. In addition, many of the non-intestinal symptoms reported by IBS sufferers are also common to those who are suffering from depression. Depression can be successfully treated with medication and lifestyle changes, so if you have any reason to suspect that depression is contributing to, or causing, your IBS symptoms to flare up, consult your doctor.

YOU REALLY NEED TO KNOW

◆ Anal bleeding is not in itself a symptom of IBS, but may be caused by piles or an anal fissure arising from constipation.

◆ Continuous bleeding from the anus is never a symptom of IBS and should be investigated by a doctor; it can be a symptom of a more serious disorder.

◆ Seemingly unrelated symptoms, from sexual difficulties to shortness of breath, could be associated with IBS symptoms.

Related problems

The digestive system

DID YOU KNOW?

Food can take two to three days to pass through the entire digestive system.

The small intestine is about 20 feet in length.

A brief look at the digestive system and at the workings of the bowel in particular will help explain how the symptoms of IBS occur.

The digestive tract

The bowel forms part of the digestive tract, a long, muscular tube that runs from the mouth to the anus and forms the body's system for taking in and breaking down food, absorbing the nutrients it provides, and disposing of the leftover waste. The internal walls of the tract are protected from general wear and tear by a coating of

SECTIONS OF THE DIGESTIVE TRACT

The digestive tract is divided into several sections, each of which has a specialized function. These are, from top to bottom: the esophagus, the stomach, the small intestine (comprised of three sections—the duodenum, the jejunum, and the ileum), and the large intestine (which includes the cecum, colon, and rectum). Together these organs make up the digestive system. The liver, gall bladder, and pancreas are also important in the process of digestion, since they supply the chemicals that help the bowel break down food.

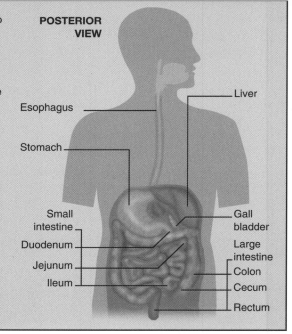

POSTERIOR VIEW

Esophagus

Stomach

Small intestine

Duodenum

Jejunum

Ileum

Liver

Gall bladder

Large intestine

Colon

Cecum

Rectum

slippery mucus, which also helps food slide along smoothly. The job of the digestive tract is to propel the food we eat from mouth to anus, allowing the body to absorb and digest nutrients along the way.

How food is digested

As we chew food, it becomes mixed with saliva, allowing it to be swallowed. The chewed food enters the throat and is pushed down through the esophagus by rhythmic contractions until it reaches the stomach. Over a period of several hours, it is broken down by acidic gastric juices into protein, starch, fat, and sugar; complex fats and sugars are also broken down here.

When the food is reduced to a semiliquid state, contractions of the stomach's muscular walls push it down into the small intestine. Here what remains of our meal is further digested, this time by alkaline juices, chemicals from the liver, gall bladder, and pancreas, and colonies of friendly bacteria.

Absorption of nutrients

By the time it reaches the end of the small intestine, the food has been reduced to a few simple chemicals. Nutrients are absorbed into the body through the walls of the small intestine, and the leftover slurry is pushed on into the large intestine.

Waste disposal

As the leftovers pass through the large intestine, water and salts are absorbed into the body through its walls. By the time the waste matter arrives in the rectum, it has become a soft, solid material ready to be expelled during the next bowel movement.

YOU REALLY NEED TO KNOW

◆ The bowel's job is to propel food from mouth to anus, allowing the body to absorb nutrients along the way.

◆ Nutrients are absorbed into the body through the walls of the small intestine.

◆ The large intestine turns leftover liquid waste into soft, solid feces (stools).

The digestive system

What causes IBS?

IBS is a real physical disorder, though the causes are not fully understood.

Stress and anxiety can worsen symptoms of IBS.

IBS does not arise from any damage to the bowel.

The symptoms of IBS are caused by changes in the way the bowel works. In IBS the bowel is found to be completely normal on examination, but it behaves abnormally from time to time. For this reason, doctors classify IBS as a "functional disorder" to distinguish it from "organic disorders" such as inflammatory bowel disease, in which there is an abnormality—an inflammation or obstruction—in part of the intestine.

Triggers

It is unclear why the bowel should misbehave in these ways in people with IBS. It may be that IBS is triggered by different things in different people. Known triggers include lack of dietary fiber, food intolerance, infections,

DIGESTION IN IBS SUFFERERS

Any disruption to the regular contractions that propel digested food through the large intestine can result in the symptoms of IBS. The nature of the disruption determines which of the possible symptoms will be experienced.

SYMPTOM	CAUSE
DIARRHEA	Contents of large intestine are pushed through too quickly, so there is not enough time for water to be removed.
CONSTIPATION	Contents of large intestine are pushed through too slowly, so too much water is extracted.
ABDOMINAL PAIN	Walls of intestine suddenly contract in spasms.

A NERVE DISORDER

IBS is a disorder in the way in which the nerves that link the brain and bowel work; this is the key to understanding the condition. The gut becomes hypersensitive, behaving exactly as in "normal" people, but with less provocation. For example, many people suffer diarrhea because of the adrenalin release associated with a job interview; in an IBS sufferer, even the small amount of adrenalin associated with a shopping trip could cause the same result. The sensations sufferers receive from their bowel may be more intense than those experienced by non-sufferers. Research shows that some individuals with IBS feel discomfort and pain when their rectums are less full of stool than would cause the same symptoms in a non-sufferer. Unfortunately, we still do not know for sure what causes this hypersensitivity.

YOU REALLY NEED TO KNOW

◆ The symptoms of IBS are caused by a malfunction in the way the bowel works—not by disease. In IBS, the bowel appears to be healthy.

◆ It is not known for sure why the bowel malfunctions in people with IBS, but certain things are known to trigger the symptoms.

antibiotics, stress, menstruation, and smoking. Because IBS is a disorder of the digestive system, many people believe that the role of food is crucial.

A real illness

Until recently, the fact that IBS sufferers appeared physically healthy led the medical profession to believe that their symptoms were due to psychological problems. Doctors believed that the personality of sufferers led them to misinterpret normal fluctuations in bowel function as symptoms of disease. This view is becoming less common. Most experts now believe that the symptoms of IBS result from a real physical malfunction.

What causes IBS?

Lack of fiber

Fiber is the part of our food that we cannot digest. Fruit and vegetables and grains such as wheat, rye, rice, and millet are all rich in fiber. Fiber is an important part of our diet because it passes through the digestive system into the large intestine, where it makes the stools bulkier. This speeds their passage through the intestine and into the rectum, and makes them easier to pass as stools.

Lack of fiber means that the stools are smaller and, as a result, the walls of the large intestine have to contract more tightly to propel them along. This slows down the system and results in constipation.

Why we lack fiber

The rise in the popularity of processed and "convenience" foods in recent decades has resulted in a steady fall in the amount of fiber in our diets. Many experts blame this decrease in dietary fiber for the increase in the so-called "Western" diseases. These include bowel cancer, gallstones, hemorrhoids (piles), constipation, and especially diverticulosis—a very common condition in which the bowel's mucous lining breaks through the outer muscle layers, causing outpouchings of the bowel wall and leading to symptoms similar to those of IBS.

The role of fiber in treatment

Today, fiber supplements, known as bulking agents, are an established part of IBS treatment. Certainly many people with IBS find that increasing their intake of dietary fiber helps their symptoms. However, others find too much fiber or the wrong type can make things worse. Many people find they are unable to tolerate gluten, a protein in wheat bran, the most common form of fiber in the Western diet (see p. 23).

THE REDISCOVERY OF FIBER

Scientific interest in the role of fiber in bowel problems was sparked by research carried out in Africa in the early 1970s. Bowel problems were known to be far less common among Africans living in rural areas, who ate a diet naturally rich in fiber and low in refined and processed foods, than they were in the industrial societies of the Western world. The researchers found that, compared to typical Americans or Europeans, the rural Africans had a faster digestive process and heavier stools.

Scientists investigating the effects of bran and other forms of dietary fiber then found that it reduced constipation, and fiber became the watchword for those who wished to eat a healthy diet.

The current recommended fiber intake for adults is 18 grams a day. This amount can be provided by two slices of whole-wheat bread, a 4-ounce portion of baked beans, and a large (6-ounce) apple, orange, or banana.

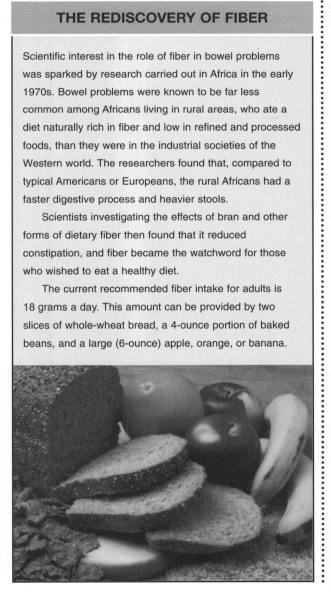

YOU REALLY NEED TO KNOW

◆ An adequate intake of fiber can help with the symptoms of IBS.

◆ Most people eat only two-thirds of the recommended daily intake of 18 grams of fiber a day.

◆ Processed and convenience foods tend to be low in fiber.

Lack of fiber

Food intolerance

Some sufferers from IBS find that certain foods trigger their symptoms.

Not all sensitivities to food are caused by an allergic reaction.

When people find that a specific type of food disagrees with them, they often say they are allergic to it. People with IBS frequently say their symptoms are triggered or at least made worse by certain foods and drinks.

This is possible, but an allergy is not to blame. An allergy is a physical reaction that results when the body's immune system attacks a foreign substance. Asthma and eczema are common conditions involving allergic reactions. To date, researchers have not been able to find such a reaction with IBS. The problem is therefore a food intolerance rather than an allergy.

How foods may trigger symptoms

There are many theories about how certain foods could cause the symptoms of IBS in some people in the absence of an allergic reaction. One theory suggests that

PROBLEM FOODS AND DRINKS

Diarrhea is one of the symptoms that can be caused by intolerance to the following foods and drinks:

◆ caffeine-containing drinks such as coffee, tea, and colas

◆ chocolate

◆ dairy products: milk, soft cheese, yogurt, ice cream

◆ fruit juices and fruit drinks

◆ sugar-free gum and mints containing sorbitol or mannitol

◆ dates and figs

◆ nuts

the symptoms of IBS may be a reaction to potentially toxic substances found in everyday food, such as the flavor-enhancer monosodium glutamate (MSG), caffeine, additives such as tartrazine, and the chemicals tyramine and histamine, both found in cheese.

Chemicals known as enzymes are produced by the digestive system to break down these substances and render them harmless. Some researchers believe that people with IBS produce fewer of such enzymes, leaving them vulnerable to the toxic effects of these substances.

The role of food intolerance in IBS remains controversial. In general, gut-stimulating foods will have a greater effect on IBS sufferers than on nonsufferers, with caffeine the worst offender. Cutting out such foods may improve symptoms for many people (see pp. 50–53).

Lactose intolerance

Those affected by lactose intolerance, which is caused by an enzyme deficiency, do not produce enough of the enzyme lactase which is needed to digest lactose, a sugar found in milk. Lactose intolerance results in IBS-like symptoms of diarrhea, stomach pain, bloating, and gas.

Celiac disease

People with celiac disease cannot tolerate gluten, a protein found in cereals such as wheat, barley, rye, and oats. This interferes with the proper digestion of food, leading to malnourishment. Symptoms usually improve quickly on a gluten-free diet.

Celiac disease may not be identified until adulthood. 70% of sufferers are women. Some of its symptoms are similar to those of IBS, but new tests have made it much easier to confirm the diagnosis.

YOU REALLY NEED TO KNOW

◆ Certain common foods may cause or worsen symptoms of IBS.

◆ The reaction to the problem food is not an allergy, since it does not involve the immune system.

◆ Food intolerances such as lactose intolerance and celiac disease can cause IBS-like symptoms, so a proper diagnosis is essential.

Food intolerance

Infections and drugs

Do consult your physician if you experience side effects from any medicines.

Don't stop taking antibiotics because of side effects, or the infection they are meant to treat could recur. If side effects are worrying you, call your doctor.

The symptoms of IBS can sometimes be caused by an illness affecting the bowels, the treatment given to cure it, or drugs given for other conditions.

Infections

Many cases of IBS seem to start after a bout of gastroenteritis or "Montezuma's revenge," which is usually caused by a bacterial infection. The invading bacteria can upset the balance of microorganisms in the bowel.

Antibiotics

Some people develop symptoms of IBS after taking a course of antibiotics. Antibiotics kill disease-causing bacteria. But they can also destroy microorganisms that

COMMON DRUGS THAT CAN AFFECT BOWEL FUNCTION

DRUG/INGREDIENT	PRODUCT	SYMPTOM/SIDE EFFECT
MAGNESIUM	Some antacids	Diarrhea
CODEINE	Some painkillers and cough medicines	Constipation
ASPIRIN, IBUPROFEN	Painkillers with an anti-inflammatory action	Diarrhea, abdominal pain
CAFFEINE	Some headache and hangover remedies	Diarrhea
IMIPRAMINE, NORTRIPTYLINE, ETC.	Tricyclic antidepressants	Constipation

Common over-the-counter and prescription drugs can cause constipation, diarrhea, or abdominal pain.

live in the digestive system, upsetting the delicate bacterial balance that aids the digestion of food. There is no definitive scientific evidence as yet that antibiotics cause IBS, and the connection has still to be proved.

Other drugs

Various other drugs can affect the way in which the bowel works. If you develop IBS symptoms while taking any drug, whether prescribed by your doctor or bought over the counter, read the information on side effects in the accompanying leaflet or on the package to see whether it could be causing the problem. If in doubt, consult your doctor or pharmacist. Never discontinue prescribed drugs without your doctor's advice.

The effects of drugs are not always clear-cut. Tricyclic antidepressants, which can cause constipation in some people, can also be an excellent treatment for some IBS sufferers (see p. 44).

(see p. 44).

YOU REALLY NEED TO KNOW

◆ Certain infections and drugs affect the bowel and may cause symptoms of IBS.

◆ You should consult your doctor if you experience any side effects as a result of taking prescribed or over-the-counter drugs.

Infections and drugs

Other causes

Stress has a direct effect on the digestive tract, causing its muscles to tense and the blood flow to increase.

Non-IBS sufferers may experience bowel disturbance when they are under stress.

Other factors besides diet, illness, and drugs can cause or worsen the symptoms of IBS. These include stress, menstruation, and smoking cigarettes.

Stress

It is unlikely that stress by itself causes IBS, but many sufferers say that their symptoms are aggravated during periods of anxiety and tension. This is hardly surprising, since we know that stress can have a powerful effect on the functioning of the bowels.

When we experience a stressful event, powerful chemicals are produced in the body—the so-called "fight or flight" hormones, of which adrenaline (epinephrine) is the best known. These ready the body for action. They prompt rapid breathing to fill the blood with oxygen and increase the heart rate and blood pressure in order to speed the freshly oxygenated blood to the muscles.

Many people faced with a stressful work situation can suffer a bout of diarrhea. Learning a relaxation technique can help avoid aggravating your IBS symptoms (see pp. 72–75).

The "fight or flight" hormones also have a direct effect on the digestive system, making the bowel contract more rapidly. This can result in a feeling of churning or "butterflies" in the stomach and, in especially alarming circumstances, sudden diarrhea.

Many people with IBS find that self-help to reduce their stress levels eases or even banishes their symptoms.

Female sex hormones

Many women with IBS find their symptoms are worse during their periods. The reason is unclear, although it is thought to be an effect of the female sex hormones, estrogen and progesterone, on the digestive system.

Research also suggests that the speed at which the bowel contracts to move food along varies at different stages of the menstrual cycle as the relative levels of these two hormones alter. In the second half of the menstrual cycle (following ovulation), food can take up to twice as long to pass through the intestine.

Some researchers have noted a connection between IBS and hysterectomy (surgical removal of the womb); 10 percent of women who have a hysterectomy go on to develop IBS symptoms. However, this may be due to the antibiotics given after the operation to prevent infection rather than the effect of surgery on hormone levels or on bowel function.

Smoking

Nicotine can interfere with the working of the bowel. It has a direct effect on the nerves controlling bowel-wall contractions and can alter their natural pattern. Many people with IBS find that smoking or sitting in a smoky atmosphere makes their symptoms worse.

YOU REALLY NEED TO KNOW

◆ Stress alone probably doesn't cause IBS, but it can make the symptoms worse.

◆ The female hormones estrogen and progesterone affect the digestive system.

Chapter

2

DIAGNOSIS & TREATMENT

Consulting your doctor

Keep a detailed record of your symptoms for a week or more before consulting your physician—this will help him or her to make a diagnosis.

Don't hesitate to ask your doctor questions if there's anything you don't understand or are worried about.

When you consult a physician about your symptoms of IBS, his or her first concern will be to make sure you do not have a more serious bowel disorder. This is because problems such as inflammatory bowel disease and cancer can cause similar symptoms to those of IBS.

What will my doctor need to know?

Your doctor will ask you about your medical history and symptoms, including how long you have been experiencing them and how often, and will give you a thorough physical examination and do some blood tests.

What examinations will be carried out?

If you are under 45 and have not unexpectedly lost weight recently, your doctor will probably keep investigations to a minimum.

The doctor will examine your abdomen with his or her hands. In IBS this normally does not reveal anything unusual apart from a slight tenderness.

The doctor will also carry out a rectal examination using a gloved index finger and a water-based lubricating gel. This can be slightly uncomfortable but it is not painful. In IBS the rectum will appear completely normal, so this examination is mainly to rule out other, more serious conditions, including cancer.

A blood sample will be taken and checked for such problems as infections and anemia.

What is normal bowel function?

In asking about your symptoms, your doctor is trying to establish whether your bowel function is normal. Normal bowel function varies greatly from one person to another and also for any individual at different times. Anything

GUIDELINES FOR DIAGNOSIS

Several characteristic symptoms known as the Manning criteria are used to diagnose IBS and distinguish it from other bowel disorders. They state that, in order to make a diagnosis of IBS, there must be at least three months' continuous or recurrent abdominal pain or discomfort that is:

◆ eased by bowel movement

◆ and/or associated with a change in frequency of bowel movement

◆ and/or associated with a change in stool consistency.

In addition, two or more of the following must apply on at least a quarter of all bowel movements or days:

◆ altered frequency of bowel movement

◆ altered stool form (that is, lumpy/hard or loose/watery)

◆ altered stool passage (straining, urgency, or a feeling of incomplete evacuation)

◆ passage of mucus

◆ a feeling of bloating.

from three or more bowel movements a week to one or two a day is considered normal. The form and consistency of the stools is also important; small, separate hard lumps ("rabbit pellets") and mushy or watery stools are both considered abnormal.

YOU REALLY NEED TO KNOW

◆ Your doctor will need to rule out the possibility of other bowel conditions before making a diagnosis of IBS.

◆ You may have to have a painless internal examination and a blood test.

◆ A diagnosis of IBS cannot be made unless the symptoms have persisted for at least three months.

Special tests

IBS symptoms are most likely to develop between the ages of 20 and 40. That is why if you are over 40 your doctor might suspect another condition.

There is currently no specific test for IBS, so these tests serve only to rule out other conditions.

If you are over 40 and your symptoms have begun recently, the doctor will take special precautions to eliminate more serious conditions than IBS. You may be asked to undergo a colonoscopy, which requires intravenous sedation. A colonoscopy is an internal examination of your bowel with a special viewing instrument. Your doctor will also perform laboratory tests to check for blood in the stools.

Any of the tests described below may be used in addition to abdominal and rectal examinations to diagnose IBS. Most people with IBS appear to be healthy. So if the results are negative, don't worry; it simply means you have IBS and not anything more serious.

Occult blood test

The word occult means "hidden"—and this test is used to check for the presence of hidden blood in the stools. It is a routine way for screening for the early signs of bowel cancer. A small amount of stool is spread onto paper that has been impregnated with one of several chemicals that react with blood by changing color.

Brushing your teeth too hard the night before can produce a positive result because it can make your gums bleed, and if you swallow the blood, traces of it may be picked up by the test. Eating lightly cooked red meat, which contains blood, can produce a similar effect. Because of these possibilities for confusion, the test is normally repeated several times to confirm the result.

Stool culture

If you are suffering from recurrent diarrhea or have had diarrhea for a prolonged period, normally more than two weeks, this test will be carried out on a sample of your

WHAT DOES IT MEAN?

OCCULT

Hidden; an occult blood test is carried out to detect blood hidden in the stools.

LACTOSE

A sugar present in milk. Some people do not produce lactase, the enzyme necessary to digest it, resulting in IBS-like symptoms, bloating, abdominal pain, flatulence, and diarrhea.

stool to check for infections. Viral infections, bacteria such as *E. coli*, *Campylobacter*, salmonella and shigella, and parasites can all lead to diarrhea. Bacterial infection is often accompanied by vomiting, however.

Lactose tolerance testing

Food intolerances in general are becoming more widespread, for reasons which are not entirely clear (see pp. 22–23). Because the symptoms of lactose intolerance are similar to those of IBS—diarrhea, pain, bloating, and gas—it may be necessary to rule out this condition before a diagnosis of IBS can be made.

Lactose intolerance is easily demonstrated by measuring breath hydrogen after consuming 2 ounces of lactose. This painless, reliable test, which can be done in your doctor's office, is based on the fact that hydrogen is released by colonic bacteria from unabsorbed lactose. It is a simple matter for your doctor to detect hydrogen on your breath.

YOU REALLY NEED TO KNOW

◆ Your doctor may recommend additional tests if you are over 40, your symptoms have started recently, or you have lost a lot of weight.

◆ The tests are intended to rule out the possibility of a more serious condition.

◆ If you have IBS, the test results will be negative.

Special tests

Examining the bowel

DOs AND DON'Ts

✔ Do follow all instructions about what to eat and drink before a test, or the result may be inconclusive and the test may have to be carried out again.

✘ Don't worry if you have to undergo these tests— they can be a bit uncomfortable, but they are not painful.

Sigmoidoscopy

The most commonly used internal examination of the bowel is a sigmoidoscopy. It allows the doctor to examine the inner walls of the lower part of the large intestine, known as the sigmoid colon. The instrument used is a sigmoidoscope, a long narrow viewing tube with a light at the tip.

The sigmoidoscope is gently inserted through your anus and rectum and into the bowel. It pumps air ahead of itself to spread the walls of the bowel apart as it moves along. The process is uncomfortable but not painful. However, the air pumped into the bowel can sometimes trigger IBS-like symptoms of pain and bloating.

Colonoscopy

This procedure is similar to a sigmoidoscopy, but the instrument used is longer and more flexible, allowing the doctor to inspect higher up the large intestine. It is very commonly done where IBS is suspected. You will be

Coating the inside of the bowels with a solution of barium sulfate means that they will show up clearly on an X-ray image.

asked to take a laxative 10–14 hours before the investigation, to clean out the bowel, and will usually be given a sedative just before the procedure.

Barium enema

A routine method used in examinations for IBS, this test takes place in a hospital radiology department. The bowels do not show up on an X-ray, so an enema is given to coat the inside of the bowel with barium sulfate, a substance that the X-ray can pick up.

You will be asked to eat nothing the night before and to take a laxative to clean out the bowel. A small amount of barium solution will be pumped gently into your bowel via a tube inserted in your anus; X-rays are then taken.

Most of the barium solution will be expelled during your next bowel movement, but your stools may be chalky white for the next couple of days. It is important to expel the barium as quickly as possible since it can worsen constipation; taking a mild laxative can help.

Ultrasound

If gallstones are suspected, ultrasound will be used. It is a completely painless and noninvasive procedure in which a special probe is passed over the outside of your abdomen. The probe emits very high frequency sound waves that bounce back off the various internal organs. A computer analyzes the returning sound waves and creates a picture of the internal organs on a screen.

Proctoscopy

Your doctor will carry out this test to detect hemorrhoids. A small instrument called a speculum is used to inspect the walls of the rectum for inflammation or bleeding.

YOU REALLY NEED TO KNOW

◆ It may be necessary to carry out a more thorough investigation of your bowel than the rectal examination done by your doctor.

◆ These tests will be carried out in your doctor's office or in a nearby hospital.

Examining the bowel

Aims of treatment

Learn as much about your condition as you can, so you can communicate with your doctor and work together to reduce your symptoms.

Be prepared to make lifestyle changes to keep your IBS under control.

IBS cannot be cured, nor do we know what causes it in all but a minority of cases. Treatments for IBS, therefore, aim either to relieve the symptoms, to prevent them from recurring, or at least reduce their severity in the long term. Some treatments succeed in doing both. Eating more fiber, for example, may provide immediate relief from constipation; if the change to the diet is permanent, it may also prevent the constipation from recurring.

Medical treatments

Drugs can certainly help alleviate diarrhea and constipation, but they are only a short-term solution. All drugs have side effects, and some of these can, in the long run, make IBS symptoms worse. Nevertheless, a short course of drug therapy can give IBS sufferers "breathing space" in which they can make changes to their diet and lifestyle to achieve a long-term improvement. For those concerned about the side effects of drugs, herbal medicine can offer a viable alternative (see p. 54).

When IBS symptoms are severe, drugs to treat constipation or diarrhea may be the best solution for short-term relief.

A CHRONIC CONDITION

Irritable bowel syndrome tends to be a long-term problem for many sufferers. It is what is known as a "chronic" condition. Examples of other chronic conditions are asthma and eczema. The term chronic condition is used to describe an illness or symptom that continues for a long period of time. The symptoms are intermittent, and there may be occasions when there is very little evidence of them at all.

A flare-up of IBS may mean that instead of the odd bout of diarrhea or constipation and the occasional spasm of pain, you suddenly begin to suffer severe symptoms, on a daily basis—severe enough to interfere with daily life. Some people with IBS lead perfectly normal lives most of the time, only to find themselves virtually housebound when the condition flares up.

Lifestyle changes

For many people, lifestyle changes are preferable to drugs for the long-term control of IBS symptoms.

Some people find that a change in diet is all that is needed to reduce or even banish their symptoms. As a general rule, a healthy balanced diet rich in fiber is best. If a food intolerance is exacerbating symptoms, it will be necessary to identify and eliminate the culprit food.

Therapies that help to reduce stress are often extremely beneficial in IBS. Counseling, psychotherapy, hypnotherapy, and relaxation techniques such as yoga, meditation, and aromatherapy can all be effective in reducing stress levels (see pp. 56–63).

YOU REALLY NEED TO KNOW

◆ There are many drugs available that can treat the symptoms of IBS, but they may cause problems in the long term.

◆ Lifestyle changes such as improving diet or reducing stress levels may be the best option for long-term control of symptoms.

Aims of treatment

Treatment for constipation

Four main types of laxatives are used to help treat constipation: bulking agents, stool softeners, osmotic agents, and stimulant laxatives.

TYPES OF LAXATIVES

TYPE	WHAT THEY ARE
BULKING AGENTS Natural bran Polycarbophil Methylcellulose Psyllium	Manufactured bulking agents are made from fiber and are taken as tablets or sprinkled on food.
STOOL SOFTENERS Docusate sodium	As the name suggests, this type of laxative softens the stools, allowing the bowel to push them along faster and making them easier to pass.

HOW THEY WORK

Bulking agents work by making the stools bulkier and softer. This allows the bowel to push them along faster and makes them easier to pass.

Stool softeners work by breaking up the surface tension of the stool. This allows it to absorb more water, making it softer.

COMMENTS

Bulking agents work slowly and gently and are the safest form of laxative to take. It is very important to drink lots of water when taking them. You will need to be patient since they can take several days to work. They are usually taken in small amounts to begin with and the dose is gradually increased until a regular pattern of bowel movement is established. Bulking agents are safe to use over extended periods of time.

Stool softeners take a day or two to work. They are given in quite large amounts at first, and these doses are reduced once the laxative begins to work.

YOU REALLY NEED TO KNOW

◆ In the long run, it is better to include more fiber in your diet than to rely on bulking agents.

◆ Bulking agents are the most suitable constipation treatment for IBS sufferers.

◆ Prolonged use of laxatives can lead to bowel damage.

◆ Liquid paraffin is sometimes used as a stool softener, but this is not advisable—it can prevent vitamin absorption, lead to serious lung problems if inhaled, and cause rectal irritation.

Treatment for constipation

Treatment for constipation

There are several types of drugs available to treat constipation, all working in different ways, and some more suitable than others for IBS sufferers.

LAXATIVES

TYPE OF LAXATIVE	WHAT THEY ARE
OSMOTIC AGENTS Magnesium sulfate Magnesium hydroxide Sodium sulfate Sodium potassium tartrate	These are salts of sodium, magnesium, or potassium; and they normally work within three hours. They include many common over-the-counter remedies for constipation.
STIMULANT LAXATIVES Bisacodyl Senna	Stimulant laxatives use irritating substances. They generally take between six and 12 hours to work and can cause cramping abdominal pain.
ENEMAS Sodium salts Phosphate Castille soap	A fluid injected through the anus into the rectum; most enemas come in a tube or bag with a nozzle applicator.

HOW THEY WORK	COMMENTS
Osmotic laxatives work by drawing large amounts of water into the large intestine to make the stools soft and loose. The water also triggers contractions that speed up the passage of the stools through the intestine.	Drink lots of water when taking osmotic laxatives to avoid dehydration. Osmotics containing sodium should not be taken by people with high blood pressure or heart, liver, or kidney problems. Osmotics containing magnesium should not be taken by people with kidney problems.
A laxative that irritates the walls of the large intestine, stimulating it to contract and propel the stools along.	Repeated use can damage the bowel or leave it unable to function properly without the laxative. Stimulant laxatives are not generally recommended for people with IBS; they make other symptoms worse.
The fluid softens and loosens any hard, dry feces stuck in the rectum.	Many substances can be used, including olive oil and simple soapy water.

YOU REALLY NEED TO KNOW

◆ You should stop taking laxatives as soon as normal bowel function is restored.

◆ Stimulant laxatives may produce a bowel movement followed by a further bout of constipation.

◆ Laxatives are not a long-term solution for constipation caused by IBS.

Treatment for constipation

Treatment for diarrhea

✓ Drink plenty of water to replace the fluids lost during a bout of diarrhea.

✗ Don't continue to take any antidiarrheal drug long-term except under medical supervision.

Many IBS sufferers will experience bouts of diarrhea, especially first thing in the morning and after meals. Taking an over-the-counter antidiarrheal drug can help control the problem, but should be regarded only as a temporary measure. To avoid dehydration, it is important to replace the fluids that are lost during a bout of diarrhea. Drink water or juice, but avoid coffee and other caffeinated drinks such as colas and tea. A drink containing salt and sugar will help to restore electrolyte balance if the diarrhea persists for a day or two. Or buy an over-the-counter oral rehydration solution that will replace sugar, salts, and other nutrients that you have lost. If you can manage to eat, try natural yogurt to restore balance to the microorganisms in your intestine

WHAT DOES IT MEAN?

BACTERIAL INFECTION
An infection by microorganisms not normally present in the body. Diarrhea is often caused by a bacterial infection in the bowel, but in IBS this is not the case.

NARCOTIC
A drug containing opium or a form of opium. Narcotics have a sedative effect and cause drowsiness, and are addictive if taken regularly.

INERT
Something that does not react chemically. Inert substances are not metabolized by the body and pass harmlessly through the digestive system.

(see p. 67). If your diarrhea persists for more than a few days, consult a doctor. (If you are elderly or you have a compromised immune system, do not wait this long.)

Types of antidiarrheal drugs

The majority of drugs used to treat diarrhea not caused by a bacterial infection fall into two categories according to how they work: those that act on the bowel wall and those that alter the contents of the bowel.

Drugs that act on the bowel wall

Opiate drugs are used to stop diarrhea and reduce the painful spasms that accompany it, which they do by slowing down the contractions of the bowel wall. This group of drugs includes loperamide (the most common ingredient in over-the-counter medications for diarrhea), diphenoxylate, and cholestyramine.

Drugs that alter bowel contents

Two types of drugs are used to relieve diarrhea by altering bowel content: bulking agents and inert powders.

Bulking agents, which are mainly used to treat constipation (see p. 38) can often make diarrhea worse, but they do work for some people, so they may be worth a try. They work by absorbing excess fluid in the large intestine. This produces larger stools, which helps the bowel return to normal. However, they may take several days to work.

Inert powders mix with the excess fluid in the large intestine and help to carry away irritating or poisonous substances. Ingredients used include calcium carbonate (chalk), charcoal, aluminum salts (such as kaolin), and pectin (made from citrus fruit).

YOU REALLY NEED TO KNOW

◆ Always consult your doctor if diarrhea lasts for more than a few days.

◆ Drugs to treat diarrhea should be seen as a temporary measure and not taken over long periods of time.

◆ Long-term use of narcotics can lead to dependence.

Treatment for diarrhea

Treating other symptoms

Some of the other symptoms of IBS, such as abdominal pain, bloating, and gas, may be sufficiently distressing to require treatment with drugs.

Antispasmodic drugs

As the name suggests, antispasmodic drugs prevent the sudden contractions of the bowel walls that cause colicky pain. They include dicyclomine and tincture of belladonna. However, many people with IBS find they are not helpful and that they cause unpleasant side effects including headaches, blurred vision, dry mouth, rashes, abdominal pain, and constipation.

Antidepressants

Some people with IBS are helped by a drug known as a tricyclic antidepressant. If your doctor suggests this to you, it does not necessarily mean that he or she thinks that your symptoms are the result of depression. Some people with IBS may indeed be depressed. However, whether their depression causes their symptoms or whether their symptoms contribute to their depression is a moot point.

The way in which tricyclic antidepressants work in IBS is not yet understood. They may work directly to reduce contractions and spasm in the walls of the bowel or on the other hand, they may decrease the amount of pain that results from these events.

Tricyclic antidepressants can produce unpleasant side effects, especially in the first week or two of treatment. These can include a dry mouth, blurred vision, and difficulty in passing urine. Unfortunately, tricyclic antidepressants can also cause constipation, which makes them unsuitable for some people with IBS.

PEPPERMINT OIL

Peppermint oil contains menthol, which has an antispasmodic effect on the bowel walls, causing them to relax. Some gastroenterologists use it during a colonoscopy (see p. 34), squirting it directly on the mucous lining of the colon to relax it so the colonoscope can be inserted further without causing discomfort. Many people with IBS find it eases symptoms of pain, gas, and particularly bloating. Peppermint oil is taken in the form of capsules that should be swallowed half an hour before meals.

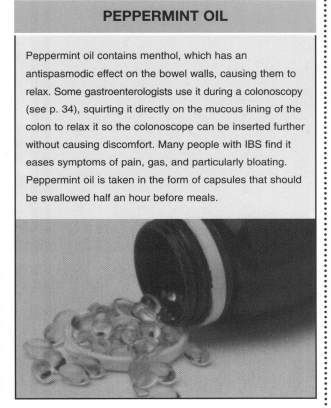

YOU REALLY NEED TO KNOW

◆ If you are suffering from severe abdominal pain, antispasmodic drugs may help in the short term; ask your physician.

◆ Antidepressants are sometimes prescribed for IBS because they relieve the physical symptoms—not because the patient is depressed.

Self-help for bloating and gas

Try drinking peppermint, chamomile, or fennel herb teas at regular intervals throughout the day. Alternatively, steep a sprig of fresh dill in a cup of boiling water for five minutes and drink the tea. Ginger can also help to reduce gas. Mix 1 teaspoon into a cup of boiling water. Prepare and drink as often as desired. Ginger can also be taken as a tincture (see Herbal treatment, pp. 54–55); add about 10 drops to any herb tea or drink.

Treating other symptoms

Chapter

3

NON-MEDICAL APPROACHES

Getting more fiber

Foods naturally rich in fiber are a better source than bran or supplements.

Not all IBS sufferers benefit from a fiber-rich diet.

Although it doesn't work for all sufferers, many people with IBS find that including more fiber in their diet helps reduce their symptoms. A high-fiber diet may also slow the progress of diverticulosis and reduce the risk of cancer of the colon, so it is therefore a sensible approach for all people with or without IBS.

How to get more fiber

The best long-term way to obtain more fiber in your diet is to eat more fiber-rich foods: fruit, vegetables, and whole grains such as brown rice and bread are all good sources of natural fiber, but you can also boost your consumption by sprinkling bran on your food or taking fiber supplements. It is important to drink plenty of water—several large glasses a day—at the same time.

Take it slowly

Don't overdo it, as this may make your symptoms worse and deter you before you feel any benefit. Make the change gradually to give your body time to adjust. If

HOW FIBER HELPS

CONSTIPATION

Fiber provides bulk for the stools, making them solid but also soft. This helps the bowel move its contents smoothly and regularly.

DIARRHEA

Additional fiber can absorb excessive fluid in the bowel and help to produce well-formed stools.

A FIBER-RICH DIET

Getting more fiber doesn't mean a radical change to your diet. Substitute fiber-rich versions for the refined foods you normally eat: whole-wheat bread instead of white, and so on. The following are ideas on adding fiber to everyday meals:

TYPICAL MEAL	FIBER-RICH VERSION
◆ Breakfast: Cornflakes, white toast with jelly, tea or coffee.	◆ Breakfast: Bran cereal, whole-wheat toast with jelly, freshly squeezed orange juice, tea or coffee.
◆ Lunch: Ham and cheese sandwich on white bread, bag of chips.	◆ Lunch: Ham and cheese sandwich with tomato and lettuce on whole-wheat bread, piece of fruit.
◆ Dinner: Chicken with white rice, frozen peas, piece of chocolate cake.	◆ Dinner: Chicken with brown rice, frozen peas, and steamed broccoli, apple cobbler made with whole-wheat flour.

increasing your fiber intake does make some symptoms worse at first, try to stick with it. Most people find that these problems go away after two or three weeks and that, gradually, over the following months, their bowel movements become regular and their other symptoms improve significantly. It is important to be patient.

YOU REALLY NEED TO KNOW

◆ Increasing your fiber intake can be particularly helpful if the main problem is constipation.

◆ It is best to increase your fiber intake gradually, and allow plenty of time for any improvement in symptoms to appear.

Getting more fiber

Problem foods

✓ Gluten intolerance, or celiac disease, is a disorder in its own right, resulting from a physical defect in the intestine.

✗ Do not assume that foods labeled "no added sugar" are sugar-free—they may contain natural sugars that can cause symptoms of IBS.

If eating more fiber makes your symptoms worse and things do not improve within two or three weeks it may be because, like many people with IBS, you are unusually sensitive to certain foods.

A minority of IBS sufferers have a food intolerance—that is, their bodies are unable to cope with certain foods. Celiac disease is an example of this. In most cases, however, IBS symptoms are not a result of food intolerance, but simply an exaggeration of the normal effects of food in the hypersensitive bowel. For example, caffeine stimulates the bowel in most people, but in an IBS sufferer it may cause diarrhea and abdominal pain.

Cutting out foods

Eliminating a problem food may be all that is necessary to improve your symptoms, although in some cases this could mean far-reaching changes to your diet.

When cutting out foods, do so for only a few days. If your symptoms improve, leading you to believe that the food concerned is causing your symptoms, consult your doctor before making long-term changes to your diet.

Gluten intolerance

A minor percentage of people with a diagnosis of IBS are in fact suffering from celiac disease (see p. 22) and are unable to tolerate gluten, a protein in many cereals including wheat, oats, barley, and rye. It may be worth cutting gluten out of your diet for a few days to see whether your symptoms improve. A gluten-free diet does not always produce a rapid improvement in symptoms, so the experiment may be inconclusive. If you still suspect that gluten is the problem, talk to your doctor, who may refer you for special antibody tests.

"Gassy" foods

If you are troubled by bloating and gas, try avoiding lentils, cabbage, and other "gassy" foods. In a vegetarian diet, however, legumes are an important source of protein. One way to reduce their "gassy" effect is to soak them well—preferably overnight—before cooking.

Sorbitol

Many people with IBS find that the artificial sweetener sorbitol, often used in diabetic or low-calorie foods and in sugar-free chewing gum, triggers their symptoms.

Natural sugars

Fructose, a fruit sugar, is another common ingredient that some people find troublesome. Lactose, a sugar found in milk, can also cause IBS-type symptoms.

TOP TEN PROBLEM FOODS

A study of patients with food intolerances, carried out at Addenbrooke's Hospital in Cambridge, England, ranked problem foods according to the percentage of patients who suffered a reaction. The top ten foods were:

FOOD	%	FOOD	%
Wheat	60	Coffee	33
Corn	44	Rye	30
Milk	44	Eggs	26
Cheese	39	Tea	25
Oats	34	Citrus fruits	24

YOU REALLY NEED TO KNOW

◆ Some IBS sufferers experience a great improvement in symptoms when they cut out problem foods.

◆ Some of the most common problem foods play a major part in our diet. Wheat flour is used in most bread, cookies, cakes, pasta, and breakfast cereals.

Problem foods

Elimination diets

A number of IBS sufferers find that certain foods or drinks trigger their symptoms. If this is the case for you, removing the offending substance may reduce the frequency of your symptoms.

Is food really the cause?

The link between IBS and food intolerance is controversial. Some sufferers undoubtedly have food intolerances; others are highly sensitive to foods that stimulate the bowel and will do well to avoid them. However, some studies have shown that secretly re-introducing foods into the diets of IBS sufferers after they have identified them as triggering symptoms does not cause a deterioration in their condition.

A sense of perspective

It is important to keep problem foods in perspective. The majority of IBS sufferers are not food intolerant, although they may feel better if they don't eat foods that stimulate the bowel. It is not always necessary to eliminate a food completely—just reducing your intake may help. With milk, for example, some people find that they can tolerate a little in tea or coffee, while drinking a glass of milk would lead to an abrupt attack of diarrhea. For some sufferers, just reviewing their diet in the light of healthy eating guidelines can help.

Identifying problem foods

Start by keeping a detailed food and drink diary for a couple of weeks. This may seem tedious, but the information it provides will be worth the effort. At the same time, keep a record of your symptoms—every bowel movement, the consistency of the stools, whether you had pain and, if so, how much (try rating pain on a scale of one to ten). Keep a record of your emotional state and menstrual cycle, too, to check whether your symptoms are affected by your mood. At the end of two weeks, you should have a good idea of which foods, if any, are producing symptoms.

Eliminating problem foods

Once you have identified the potential culprit, cut it out of your diet for a few days and then re-introduce it back in. Make a careful note of your symptoms before and after removing a particular food and after re-introducing it. This is known as a simple elimination or exclusion diet.

If you have identified more than one troublesome food, do not cut them out without professional advice, or you may be exchanging your IBS symptoms for nutritional deficiencies.

SEEKING PROFESSIONAL HELP

If you think your symptoms are being caused by a number of foods, seek professional help before drastically reducing your diet. Your physician can refer you to a dietician or nutritionist. You may have to go on a multiple exclusion or restriction diet, more complex versions of the simple exclusion diet in which several potentially troublesome foods are removed, and re-introduced one by one.

If you find that you have a food intolerance or are sensitive to several foods, your dietician will help you to find good alternatives so you can still eat a balanced and healthy diet.

YOU REALLY NEED TO KNOW

◆ Eliminating foods to which you are sensitive may reduce your symptoms.

◆ Seek professional advice before eliminating foods in the long term so you can still eat a healthy, balanced diet.

Herbal treatment

Herbal medicine can be extremely helpful to IBS sufferers. Some herbal remedies have direct beneficial effects on the digestive system, and, taken under the supervision of a qualified medical herbalist, they have few, if any, unwanted side effects. It is important in chronic conditions like IBS, in which symptoms may come and go for years, to have "safe" treatment at hand to deal with them as and when they arise.

Consult a professional

It is important to make a distinction between the treatment offered by a professional medical herbalist and over-the-counter herbal remedies. A herbalist will examine you and discuss your overall state of health, physical and emotional, as well as your IBS symptoms, before prescribing a remedy tailor-made for your needs.

Some people find that prepackaged herbal remedies help ease their IBS symptoms—everyone is different, and it may be worth trying some to find out. Generally, however, professional treatment is more effective.

A word of warning

Although herbal remedies are popularly regarded as gentle alternatives to conventional medicines, herbs are powerful substances and can be dangerous if misused. Taking a prepackaged remedy will be safe enough if you follow the instructions, but never try to make your own remedies—always seek professional help.

Herbal preparations

The most familiar preparation is an infusion, or "tea"; the fresh or dried leaves or flowers of the plant are steeped in hot water for about 15 minutes, then the liquid is drained off and drunk. Decoctions (made by a similar method, but from hard parts of a plant, such as roots, seeds, and bark) and tinctures (a mixture of water and alcohol in which herbs have been soaked) are more complicated to prepare and are best obtained from a herbalist.

HERBAL REMEDIES FOR IBS

SYMPTOMS	REMEDY
PAINFUL SPASMS, BLOATING, GAS	Peppermint, chamomile, or fennel, taken in infusion. Take any time. Avoid high doses of fennel during pregnancy.
PAINFUL SPASMS	Valerian: soak 1 teaspoon of powder in a tall glass of water overnight, or take tincture or tablets. Take any time. Wild yam: infusion of 1 teaspoon with 1 pint water, or take tincture or tablets. Avoid when pregnant.
DIARRHEA, NAUSEA	Slippery elm: mix 1 teaspoon of powder in a tall glass of water or take capsules. Take three times daily before meals.

YOU REALLY NEED TO KNOW

◆ Herbal treatment may relieve the symptoms of IBS without the side effects associated with drugs.

◆ You should not undertake self-treatment with herbs; consult a qualified medical herbalist.

Herbal treatment

Talking therapies

SELF-HELP

Keep a record of your symptoms and emotional state to see if a pattern emerges.

Do not talk to family or friends if it makes you uncomfortable—your doctor will be able to recommend a counselor.

You may find that your symptoms are triggered or worsened by periods of stress and tension. This is not really surprising. Stress and anxiety can cause bowel symptoms in most people, and all the more so in IBS sufferers, where the bowel is hypersensitive.

IBS is associated with anxiety, and sufferers continually score higher on scales designed to measure anxiety levels. It is also associated with depression and "illness attitudes" such as hypochondria and disease phobia. For some sufferers, therefore, counseling and psychotherapy can address these problems and help to reduce symptoms.

How do they work?

At their simplest, these therapies can help you find ways to tackle difficult problems and so reduce the stress that is contributing to your symptoms. Psychotherapy can

STRESS AND IBS SYMPTOMS

The relationship between stress and IBS symptoms can be a circular one. Stress, whatever its cause, may cause symptoms to flare up, leaving the sufferer feeling unable to cope with life, particularly if symptoms are severe. The resulting sense of losing control over life can exacerbate stress, starting the cycle all over again.

Stress

Worsening of symptoms

Reduced ability to cope

Feelings of helplessness

also help identify and resolve deeper areas of emotional conflict that manifest themselves in physical symptoms, although you may not be conscious of them day to day.

Counseling

A counselor can provide a sympathetic and practical listening ear in a safe environment, allowing you to talk about and address your problems.

We have all experienced the relief of talking over a particularly worrying problem with a good friend. Talking through a problem is the first step toward dealing with it or, if that is not possible, accepting it and moving on.

Sometimes we can deal with problems by discussing them with family and friends. However, it is not always easy to discuss personal problems—marital difficulties, for example—with a close family member or friend without involving them in distress and worry. It can be better to have a listener who is not as emotionally close as our family and friends and can give objective advice. This is what a counselor does.

Psychotherapy

Like counselors, psychotherapists talk with their patients. This form of counseling explores the individual's deep-seated, and often subconscious, conflicts and emotions, examining their effect on his or her everyday life. Psychotherapists may work with the people who consult them by using methods such as role play, helping to identify and understand their underlying problems and find ways of solving them.

Psychotherapists are not usually medically trained doctors and do not prescribe drugs. They are often social workers or psychologists.

YOU REALLY NEED TO KNOW

◆ Counselors lend a sympathetic, objective, and practical listening ear to address your problems.

◆ Psychotherapy helps identify and resolve subconscious conflicts that can produce physical symptoms.

Talking therapies

Hypnotherapy

✓ Hypnotherapy has been approved as a useful medical tool by the American Medical Association since 1958.

✗ You cannot be made to act against your will while you are in a hypnotic trance.

Hypnotherapy, the healing of a person while they are in a trancelike state or hypnotized, is one of the most effective treatments for IBS. Many sufferers find their symptoms improve greatly after only a short course of treatment and that the improvement lasts.

Hypnotherapy is one of the best-researched and most widely used complementary therapies. It is used in hospitals and research centers around the world to treat a wide range of health problems. In addition to IBS, hypnotherapy can treat chronic pain, migraine, many stress-related conditions, anxiety, depression, phobias, and addiction, and can reduce pain during childbirth.

How hypnotherapy works

Scientists have been trying to discover for many years exactly how hypnotherapy works. It is now thought that hypnosis puts the two sides of the brain—the left, which tends to deal with language and logic, and the right, which handles emotions and symbolism—in closer communication with each other. This allows connections between behavior and its underlying causes to be identified and understood. Whether or not this is true,

A WORD OF WARNING

Like most medical techniques, hypnosis is very safe in skilled hands. However, it is a powerful tool and can be dangerous if mishandled. For this reason it is important to consult a properly qualified practitioner, preferably a medical doctor or dentist or, failing that, someone with training in clinical psychology.

VISUALIZATION

A hypnotherapist may induce your trance by inviting you to imagine a place where you feel comfortable, a room at home, a tropical beach, or a forest glade. Think of a scene where you feel safe and able to relax.

hypnotherapy is essentially a relaxation therapy. During a hypnotic trance, the body relaxes deeply in much the same way as during meditation. The heart rate slows, breathing deepens, and blood pressure decreases. While in the trance, you are more open to suggestion, and this is the key to dealing with problems through hypnosis.

Hypnotherapy in practice

The practitioner will talk to you for a while and then ask you to imagine you are drifting or sinking into comfort. As you relax, your eyelids will begin to feel heavy and your eyes will close. You will then be in a light hypnotic trance. You will feel you are between waking and sleeping, aware of everything around you but detached from it. You can speak and end the trance whenever you wish.

Once you are in a trance, the practitioner can look for subconscious causes of your symptoms. When these have been found, he or she can suggest solutions to you, aiming to replace negative thought patterns with positive ones.

Meditation

✓ Scientific research has shown that meditation enables the body to enter a state of deep relaxation.

✗ Meditation does not have to take place in the traditional cross-legged position. You can sit any way you like, as long as your back is straight and your body is relaxed.

Research shows that daily meditation can improve both mental and physical health; many IBS sufferers find that regular meditation brings about a marked improvement in their symptoms or, in some cases, can even eliminate them altogether.

In addition to IBS, it has been shown to help with high blood pressure, chronic pain, asthma, and heart disease. During meditation the heart rate and breathing rate both decrease, and brain activity alters to patterns only seen during very deep relaxation. Those who meditate regularly have described feelings of well-being, mental clarity, and peace.

The scientific basis

Scientific investigation into the effects of meditation was pioneered in the 1960s by the American researcher Dr. Herbert Benson. He came up with the term "relaxation

LEARNING TO MEDITATE

◆ Choose a warm, comfortable room, quiet and not too bright. Take the phone off the hook. Sit comfortably on a chair or on the floor, making sure your back is straight.

◆ You may find it helps to concentrate on an object such as a candle flame, visualize a pleasant scene, or close your eyes and repeat a word or phrase in your head.

◆ Do not try to concentrate your mind; try to allow it to become empty.

◆ If your mind wanders, accept this and do not become irritated by it; just gently return your concentration to your meditation object. With practice, you will do this almost without thought.

◆ Be patient with yourself; meditation takes practice.

◆ Breathe slowly and regularly, through the nose rather than the mouth and into the abdomen rather than the chest (see p. 74).

BENEFITS OF MEDITATION

Practiced regularly, meditation can help you control some of the triggers that aggravate the symptoms of IBS, such as stress and tension by:

◆ Lowering the heart rate.

◆ Reducing blood pressure.

◆ Relaxing the muscles.

◆ Helping to alleviate insomnia.

response" to describe the physical effects of meditation and noted that these were the direct opposite of the body's adrenalin-induced "fight or flight" response—the instinctive human reaction to stress, fear, and danger—when the heart and breathing rate both increase.

Transcendental meditation

Often referred to as simply TM, transcendental meditation is the most popular form of meditation in the developed Western world. Most of the research into the health benefits of meditation has involved TM.

Practitioners of TM repeat short words or phrases (known as mantras) in their heads to help them overcome conscious thought and reach what is called a state of "deep consciousness" or "thought-free awareness." This stage transcends thought (hence the name) and allows the individual direct access to their energy and creative "center."

Meditation

Aromatherapy and yoga

DOs AND DON'Ts

✓ Do attend a yoga class at first so you can learn the postures properly.

✗ Some aromatherapy oils should not be used by those with high blood pressure, kidney disease, or during pregnancy. Check with an aromatherapist first.

Many other complementary therapies can be helpful in reducing stress, but two of the most useful for sufferers from IBS are aromatherapy and yoga.

Aromatherapy

Aromatherapy uses essential plant oils to produce therapeutic effects. The oils are extracted from the flower, buds, or root of the plant, or from the fruit peel (citrus oils). Extraction methods include distillation and expression (squeezing or pressing).

Each oil has its own characteristic aroma. Some oils have specific medicinal properties; for example, lavender is antiseptic. Others have an effect on mood—some are soothing, others are stimulating. Massaging the abdomen with essential oils is relaxing and can help to ease the symptoms of IBS.

USING ESSENTIAL OILS

Essential oils are extremely strong and are used in tiny amounts. They should be added to a much larger amount of a "carrier" oil such as wheat germ, sweet almond, or grape seed before they are used.

To prepare oils for an aromatherapy massage, add between two and five drops of essential oil to 2 teaspoons of carrier oil and shake well. The proportion of essential oil in the blend should not exceed 3 percent, whether you are using a single essential oil or a combination.

For an abdominal massage to soothe IBS symptoms, try a mixture of essential oils of peppermint and black pepper or, alternatively, rosemary and marjoram.

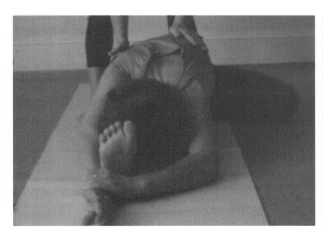

Yoga is a good overall relaxation therapy, and certain positions are reputed to aid digestion and bowel function.

Yoga

The health benefits of yoga have been researched for many years. Regular practice has been shown to reduce high blood pressure, lower levels of anxiety and stress, and promote relaxation.

An ancient Indian system of breathing and body exercises, yoga is actually a complete philosophy in itself that aims, eventually, to bring the individual into harmony with the universe. However, the vast majority of Westerners who practice yoga do it simply because it helps keep them fit and supple, and promotes a sense of well-being and relaxation.

You can teach yourself yoga from a book, but it is always better to attend a class, at least to begin with, because it is important to learn the various postures properly. For maximum benefits, it is recommended that you practice yoga on a regular basis—ideally every day—rather than just attending a class once a week.

Aromatherapy and yoga

Chapter

LIVING WITH IBS

Improving your diet

FACTS

✓ Overcooking fruit and vegetables can destroy the nutrients they contain.

✗ Avoid tea and coffee because they cause you to retain water; drink herbal tea or water instead if you want to boost your fluid intake.

Even if your IBS symptoms are not caused by a food intolerance, improving your diet may prevent them from flaring up. As a general principle, avoid processed foods and "TV dinners," which generally contain additives, and aim for a wholesome diet of fresh foods.

Whole grains

The importance of fiber to normal bowel function is well established. Choose whole-grain versions of foods rather than their refined counterparts to add fiber to your diet.

Fruits and vegetables

Eaten raw, or lightly cooked for maximum nutritional value, fruits and vegetables are excellent sources of fiber and contain essential vitamins and minerals. Eat fresh fruit between meals rather than fatty or sugary foods.

Water

Drink plenty of water. This is especially important if you are constipated, though you should also drink lots of water during bouts of diarrhea to avoid dehydration.

The human body needs at least 2½ pints (1.5 liters) of water a day—the amount shown here—to stay healthy. Drink water with meals, and sip water or herbal tea throughout the day to meet your quota.

HOW TO EAT

In a condition such as IBS, in which both diet and stress can play important roles, how you eat can be just as important as what you eat.

◆ Have small meals at regular times throughout the day—this is easier for the digestive system to handle than a lot of snacking and one big meal.

◆ Always make time for breakfast, however busy you are—if necessary, get up 15 minutes earlier in the morning.

◆ Eat a substantial lunch.

◆ Make your evening meal the lightest of the day, and eat at 7 or 8 P.M. rather than 10 P.M. to give your body time to begin digesting your food before bedtime.

◆ Never rush a meal or eat "on the run." Make time to eat in a leisurely fashion.

◆ Sit down to eat, concentrate on what you are eating, and chew food thoroughly.

YOU REALLY
NEED TO KNOW

◆ Eat a wholesome diet with plenty of fruits and vegetables—aim for five servings a day.

◆ Drink at least 2½ pints (1.5 liters) of water a day.

◆ Eat your main meal around noon, not in the evening.

Yogurt

The balance of microorganisms in the bowel can be upset by a bout of gastroenteritis or "Montezuma's revenge," triggering IBS symptoms. To help the bowel replenish the levels of healthy bacteria, try eating plenty of natural, unsweetened "live" yogurt.

The beneficial ingredient in "live" yogurt is a bacterium called *Lactobacillus acidophilus*; you can take this in the form of a daily supplement if you prefer.

Improving your diet

Foods to avoid

Some of the foods discussed here are best avoided or eaten only in limited quantities by anyone who wants to have a healthy diet. Others are mentioned because they can trigger symptoms in some IBS sufferers—you may have to experiment to see whether this is true for you.

In addition to the foods listed here, some people have intolerances (see p. 48) to "gassy" foods such as beans, lentils, brussels sprouts, peas, and cabbage, the artificial sweetener sorbitol—used extensively in so-called "diet" products and in sugar-free chewing gum—and the fruit sugar fructose.

Red meat

Many people with IBS find that eating red meat triggers their symptoms, so it may be worth cutting it out to see if this helps. Eat fish and poultry instead to make sure you are getting enough protein, and whole grains and dark green vegetables to maintain your supply of iron.

Saturated fats

Most of us eat too much fat, and saturated fat—the kind present in foods of animal origin, such as meat and dairy products—can be harmful to your health. Reduce your intake by switching from whole milk to 1% or 2% milk, or skim milk, and replacing cream with low-fat yogurt. Spread butter thinly on your bread (do not replace it with margarine, which is a highly refined product containing preservatives and additives). Eat only small amounts of cheese; about 1½ ounces (40g) daily is enough.

Foods that are fried or roasted absorb large amounts of fat, so try to keep these methods of cooking to an absolute minimum. As a general rule you should steam, broil, or bake food instead.

Spicy foods

Many people with IBS find that foods that are heavily spiced—some Indian dishes, for example—make their symptoms worse. Note your symptoms after your next meal containing spicy food to see if this applies to you.

Caffeine

Because caffeine can have a powerful effect on bowel function, it is worth cutting out tea, coffee, and colas, to see whether this helps. You will not lose out nutritionally by doing this, as long as your overall fluid intake remains adequate. Switch to water and herbal teas instead.

Alcohol

In some people alcohol can irritate the bowel, especially if drunk in excess. A glass or two of wine a day is unlikely to make much difference. However, it may be worth cutting out alcohol completely for a while to see if you are particularly sensitive to its effects. If you do drink alcohol, always accompany it with some food.

MODERATE YOUR DIET	
AVOID	**REPLACE WITH**
◆ Coffee, tea, and colas	◆ Herbal teas
◆ Whole dairy products	◆ Low-fat dairy products
◆ Red meats	◆ Fish and chicken
◆ Prepackaged and processed foods	◆ Fresh fruits and vegetables

4

YOU REALLY NEED TO KNOW

◆ The information on food packaging usually includes the saturated fat content of the food, so you can check it.

◆ Caffeine is present not only in tea and coffee, but also in chocolate and cola drinks.

Foods to avoid

Dealing with stress

Make a list of the things that cause you to become stressed and decide what you can change and what you can't.

Don't try to do it all alone; think of practical solutions for the things you can change, and enlist any support you need for those you can't.

In many cases there is a clear relationship between IBS symptoms and stress. Taking action to reduce your stress level is therefore an important step toward improving your symptoms.

Why is stress bad?

Not all stress is bad. Happy events, such as getting married or being promoted at work, can cause stress, but because we view these things in a positive way, we generally take the uncertainty they cause in stride.

Stress is an inevitable part of being alive. A life wholly without stress, where everything was predictable and no effort was ever required to deal with problems, would be a life without achievement or reward. Constant stress, however, can be harmful to your health, particularly if you feel you have no control over your situation.

Our reaction to different types of stress is highly individual. The important thing is to identify the situations you personally find stressful, change them if you can, and learn to live with them if you cannot. In order to cope better with unavoidable stresses, it is often necessary to learn to relax (see pp. 72–75) and view them in a positive rather than a negative way.

Plan to avoid stress

Each of us faces routine situations every day that make us feel "wound up." Avoidance can be the best method for removing these everyday stresses.

Reschedule your day. For example, if your route to work is difficult and you are often late, allow more time. Leave home earlier to avoid the worst of the rush hour. It will mean getting up a bit earlier, but that is a small price to pay for keeping your stress levels down.

Plan ahead. If shopping in a crowded supermarket makes your blood boil, try to do your shopping at less busy times. If you seem to end up in line for ages every single time you go to the post office, find out when the quiet periods are and then go whenever possible.

Unavoidable stress

Other sources of long-term stress, such as problems with family members, neighbors, and work colleagues, may be less easy to deal with, and ultimately you may have to learn to live with them. In this sort of complicated situation, many people find that counseling (see p. 54) can help them to understand their problems better and find, if not solutions, then ways of living with them.

MONEY WORRIES

Money is the cause of some of life's biggest stresses. A realistic view of what you need and what you can afford combined with a bit of planning ahead can go a long way toward reducing stress.

Try to budget your expenditure. Budget for bills that will be coming along in the next few months and put aside the money to pay them before they are due. If you have run up a large credit card bill, plan to pay it off in regular installments—figure out what you can afford each month and how long it will take to pay the total.

Taking control of your finances this way may seem complicated and time-consuming at first, but after the initial effort it will become much easier, and it will relieve you of a great deal of worry.

YOU REALLY NEED TO KNOW

◆ Stress plays a major role in IBS.

◆ Taking positive action to deal with problems will increase your sense of control over events and help reduce stress.

◆ Setting aside some time each day just for yourself can prevent stress from building up over time.

Dealing with stress

A less stressful lifestyle

✓ Make time for stress-reduction activities. Schedule them into your calendar and treat them with the same importance that you would treat an appointment.

✗ Don't ignore the signs that you are becoming stressed— such as irritability or sleeplessness.

Whatever the specific stresses in your life, they will be easier to deal with if you are physically fit, rested, and have a positive self-image. Some basic lifestyle changes can go a long way toward reducing your stress levels. In addition to the advice given here, a good diet and proper eating habits (see pp. 64–65) are also an important part of a stress-reducing lifestyle.

Exercise
Regular aerobic exercise can improve IBS symptoms, help you relax and sleep better, get you fit, build a better self-image, and encourage positive thinking. Aim to exercise for 20 minutes at least three times a week. Choose a form of exercise that leaves you slightly breathless, such as jogging, swimming, or cycling.

Get enough sleep
Most people need seven to eight hours of sleep a night. Get into the habit of going to bed and getting up at a regular time. Reserve your bedroom for sleeping and lovemaking—don't watch TV, eat, or work there. Avoid eating and drinking late at night; this can prevent you from sleeping properly. Ensure that your bed is comfortable.

Cut out smoking
If you smoke, try to give it up or at least to cut down. Nicotine has a powerful effect on bowel function, and quitting will help reduce your symptoms.

Drink in moderation
Many people feel that having a few drinks helps them to relax, but in the long run, the opposite is the case, particularly with excessive drinking. Too much alcohol

can irritate the bowel. Don't drink on an empty stomach. At a party or similar function, pace your drinking by alternating alcoholic drinks with glasses of water.

Relaxation

Try to put some time aside each day, even if it is only 30 minutes or so, to relax. This should be your time, a space in the day when you unwind and forget about the family, the bills, work, and all your other worries.

During this period, switch off the TV and take the phone off the hook—or turn down the volume on the answering machine—and do something that relaxes you. Have a candlelit bath, diffuse an aromatic essential oil in your bedroom and simply lie down and drift away, read a book, or take the dog for a walk—whatever works for you.

EXERCISE

Getting regular exercise can be very beneficial in relieving the symptoms of IBS. It helps to reduce stress levels, and also the discomfort of bloating and distension.

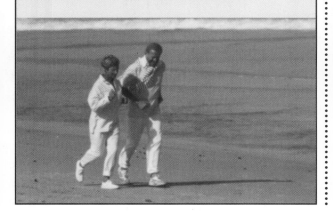

YOU REALLY NEED TO KNOW

◆ Changes in lifestyle can have a major impact on stress.

◆ Counseling, regular exercise, getting enough sleep, a healthy diet, giving up smoking, and keeping your alcohol intake down can all help.

◆ Relaxation doesn't necessarily mean doing nothing—it could be an absorbing activity that takes your mind off your worries.

A less stressful lifestyle

Breathing and relaxation

Learn to observe your chest and abdomen so you can tell whether you are breathing correctly.

Practice the breathing exercise so you can switch to relaxed breathing at will.

Breathing correctly is an important aid to handling stress. There are two ways of breathing, and the body employs them in different situations.

Relaxed breathing

When your breathing is relaxed, the diaphragm—the dome-shaped muscle that separates the chest from the abdomen—contracts, pushing the contents of the abdomen down and creating a vacuum in the chest, which causes air to be sucked into the lungs. The diaphragm then relaxes, and the contents of the abdomen rise back up, forcing air back out of the lungs.

TENSE BREATHING

When we become frightened or angry, the pattern of our breathing automatically changes. Instead of using the diaphragm, we begin to suck air into the lungs using the intercostal muscles between our ribs. This way we take quick, shallow breaths that allow us to pump the blood full of the maximum amount of oxygen in the shortest possible time. This prepares the body to either fight or flee—our instinctive response to any threat. After the danger has receded, the body automatically reverts to the relaxed diaphragm breathing.

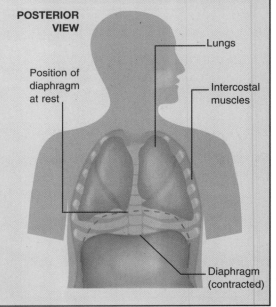

POSTERIOR VIEW

Position of diaphragm at rest

Lungs

Intercostal muscles

Diaphragm (contracted)

A SIMPLE BREATHING EXERCISE

Lie down in a quiet room. Close your eyes. Place one hand on your chest and the other on your abdomen just below the rib cage. Breathe in slowly, allowing your abdomen to push up. Breathe out and feel your abdomen flatten. This is breathing with the diaphragm—your chest should hardly move.

Breathe like this for several minutes, getting into an easy, slow rhythm, and you will feel yourself relax. When you are feeling stressed and upset, check your breathing. If you are breathing using your chest, gently correct the pattern by breathing into your abdomen.

With a bit of practice you will be able to do this anywhere—in your car in a traffic jam, at your desk, or in a supermarket check-out line.

YOU REALLY NEED TO KNOW

◆ Breathing correctly helps to reduce your stress levels.

◆ Normal, relaxed breathing uses the diaphragm, not the chest muscles.

When you breathe this way, breathing in pushes out the front of your abdomen and breathing out allows it to flatten again.

How stress affects our breathing

During periods of long-term stress and anxiety, it is often possible to get into the habit of tense incorrect breathing. This means that the body continues to run on "red alert," setting up a vicious circle of stress and tension that can eventually cause a variety of stress-induced health problems.

By becoming more aware of changes in your breathing pattern, you will be able to help yourself to relax by deliberately breathing with the diaphragm.

Breathing and relaxation

Understanding the jargon

Medicine is full of technical terms and words that can make a condition such as irritable bowel syndrome seem more daunting than it really is. Knowing what the terms mean can clarify your condition and let you communicate more easily with your doctor.

ALLERGY—a physical reaction that results when the body's immune system attacks a foreign substance. Asthma and eczema are common conditions involving allergic reactions.

ANAL FISSURE—a tear in the lining of the anal canal usually caused by passing very large, hard stools.

BARIUM ENEMA—a preparation of barium sulfate used to coat the inner bowel walls, allowing them to be examined on X-ray. It is introduced into the bowel via a tube inserted into the anus.

CELIAC DISEASE—a condition in which the body cannot tolerate gluten, a protein found in cereals such as wheat, barley, rye, and oats.

COLONOSCOPY—internal examination of the large intestine using a long, flexible viewing tube with a light at the tip (colonoscope).

CONSTIPATION—usually defined as having a bowel movement less than twice a week or straining to pass stools more than 25 percent of the time.

DIARRHEA—a loose consistency of stool with increased frequency of bowel motions.

DUODENUM—the upper part of the small intestine.

ENZYMES—chemicals produced by the digestive system to break down potentially toxic substances found in food and render them harmless.

ESOPHAGUS—the tube leading from the throat to the stomach.

FIBER—the part of our food that we cannot digest. It passes through the digestive system and makes the stools bulkier, speeding their passage through the digestive system and making them easier to pass.

FLATULENCE (GAS)—the expulsion through the anus of waste gases from the digestive system.

FUNCTIONAL DISORDER—a change in the way a bodily process works (digestion in IBS), not caused by disease.

GASTROENTERITIS—nausea, vomiting, and diarrhea caused by a bacterial infection.

GASTROENTEROLOGY—the medical science concerned with problems of the digestive system.

HEMORRHOIDS (PILES)—soft lumps that can develop in and around the anus as a result of straining to pass stools due to constipation.

ILEUM—the lowest part of the small intestine.

JEJUNUM—the middle section of the small intestine.

SYNDROME—a collection of symptoms that occur together and are associated with a single disorder.

ULTRASOUND—a non-invasive procedure that uses high-frequency sound waves to examine internal organs.

Useful addresses

IBS SUPPORT GROUP FOR SOUTHERN CALIFORNIA
6064 Magnol Lane
Woodland Hills, CA 91367
www.geocities.com

NATIONAL DIGESTIVE DISEASES CLEARINGHOUSE (NDDIC)
2 Information Way
Bethesda, MD 20892-3570
Tel: (301) 654-3810
Fax: (301) 507-8906
www.middk.gov
email: nddic@info.niddk.nih.gov

AMERICAN DIGESTIVE HEALTH FOUNDATION
7910 Woodmont Avenue
7th floor
Bethesda, MD 20814-3015
Tel: (301) 654-2635
Fax: (301) 654-1140
www.gastro.org

CELIAC SPRUE ASSOCIATION/USA
P.O. Box 31700
Omaha, NE 68131-0700
Tel: (402) 558-0600
Fax: (402) 558-1347

IBS NETWORK
www.ibsnetwork.org.uk

DIGESTIVE DISEASE NATIONAL COALITION (DONC)
507 Capitol Court NE, Suite 2007
Washington, DC 20002
Tel: (202) 544-7497
Fax: (202) 546-7105
email: info@cff.org

GLUTEN INTOLERANCE GROUP OF NORTH AMERICA (GIGNA)
P.O. Box 23053
Seattle, WA 98102-0353
Tel: (206) 325-6980
Fax: (206) 850-2394
email: gig@accessone.com

EDELSON CENTER FOR ENVIRONMENTAL & PREVENTATIVE MEDICINE
3833 Roswell Road
Suite 110
Atlanta, GA 30342
Tel: (404) 841-0088
Fax: (404) 841-6416
www.ephca.com/testibs1.htm

AMERICAN GASTRO-ENTEROLOGICAL ASSOCIATION
www.gastro.org/ibs.html

INTERNATIONAL FOUNDATION FOR FUNCTIONAL GASTROINTESTINAL DISORDERS
P.O. Box 17864
Milwaukee, WI 53217
Tel: (414) 241-9479
www.execpc.com/iffgd

INTESTINAL DISEASE FOUNDATION
1323 Forbes Avenue, Suite 200
Pittsburgh, PA 15219
Tel: (412) 261-5888
Fax: (412) 471-2722

Index

Index

Acknowledgments

SPL= Science Photo Library

Photographs: 19 Astrid & Hanns-Frieder Michler/SPL; 26 BSIP Chassenet/SPL;
28/29 Tek Image/SPL; 34 CNRI/SPL; 46/47 John Greim/SPL; 58/59 Sinclair Stammers/SPL;
63 Francoise Sauze/SPL; 64/65 BSIP, LECA/SPL; 73 Gable, Jerrican/SPL

Illustrations: Axis Design Editions Limited

This book was edited and designed by Axis Design Editions Limited,
8 Accommodation Road, London NW11 8ED